Distribution, publication, and copying in any form are prohibited and subject to damages.

TEN HYPNOSES

Copying, publishing, and sharing with third parties are only permitted with the written consent of the author. Please observe the notes on copyright and usage.

Distribution, publication, and copying in any form are prohibited and subject to damages.

Copying, publishing, and sharing with third parties are only permitted with the written consent of the author. Please observe the notes on copyright and usage.

Ingo Michael Simon

TEN HYPNOSES

12
Chronic Pain

Distribution, publication, and copying in any form are prohibited and subject to damages.

© 2024 Ingo Michael Simon
All rights reserved.
Independently published
www.ingosimon.com

Important Notes for Urgent Attention:
The contents of this book are based on the practical experiences of the author with hypnosis applications and psychotherapy in a trance state. Although the author has strived for the utmost care, errors or misunderstandings in the presentation cannot be completely excluded. Therapeutic work with people and the application of hypnosis are solely the responsibility of the hypnotist. It cannot be ruled out that parts of this book may be misunderstood or that the application of a presented procedure may cause an undesirable reaction in the client. The author also assumes no co-responsibility if work with a client is carried out with reference to the statements in this book.

The Author:
Ingo Michael Simon studied psychology and education and is a hypnotherapist with practices in southwestern Germany and Switzerland. With the help of hypnosis-supported psychotherapy, he primarily treats people with persistent psychological conditions. His practice focuses on anxiety disorders, pathological compulsions, and psychosomatic illnesses. His therapeutic offerings mainly include classical and modern hypnosis applications and the dreamland therapy he developed himself.

Copying, publishing, and sharing with third parties are only permitted with the written consent of the author. Please observe the notes on copyright and usage.

Distribution, publication, and copying in any form are prohibited and subject to damages.

Notes on Copyright and Usage

Copying, publishing, and sharing with third parties is prohibited and only permitted with the written consent of the author. Please observe the following copyright and usage guidelines.

This work has been carefully crafted and created to the best of the author's knowledge and personal experience. It comprises text templates and application guidelines for professional hypnosis sessions. The author is a licensed psychotherapist with extensive experience in psychotherapy, coaching, and personal training using hypnotic techniques and methods. Nevertheless, the author and the publisher assume no liability for the accuracy of information, instructions, and advice, nor for any typographical errors. The author and publisher accept no responsibility or liability for the application of these texts and recommendations with clients or patients, nor for any potential consequences or unexpected reactions. It is expressly noted that the application of therapeutic and advisory techniques and formulations lies solely and entirely within the responsibility of the practitioner. This also applies to adherence to the boundaries of legally regulated medical and therapeutic practices. The fact that a book containing action proposals is freely available for sale does not imply that its application with clients or patients is permitted for everyone.

Distribution, publication, and copying in any form are prohibited and subject to damages.

Copying, publishing, and sharing with third parties are only permitted with the written consent of the author. Please observe the notes on copyright and usage.

Distribution, publication, and copying in any form are prohibited and subject to damages.

Table of Contents

Introduction 9

#1 11

#2 16

#3 21

#4 26

#5 32

#6 37

#7 42

#8 48

#9 53

#10 58

Overview of All Titles in the Series "Ten Hypnoses" 63

Copying, publishing, and sharing with third parties are only permitted with the written consent of the author. Please observe the notes on copyright and usage.

Distribution, publication, and copying in any form are prohibited and subject to damages.

Copying, publishing, and sharing with third parties are only permitted with the written consent of the author. Please observe the notes on copyright and usage.

Introduction

The series "Ten Hypnoses" is very well known in Germany, Austria, and Switzerland as a collection of texts for therapeutic work and is used by numerous psychotherapeutic practices, doctors, therapists, coaches, and other helping professionals. I am pleased to now be able to offer these texts in other countries as well.

Most therapists have their own methods for inducing and deepening trance as well as for exiting trance. Therefore, I have focused on the main part of the hypnosis. The texts in this book can be integrated as the main part into any hypnosis process.

The texts in this collection use various hypnosis techniques. I will not explain these in detail, as I assume that users have the appropriate training. It is also not necessary to understand the exact structure or functioning of the different parts. The texts can simply be read aloud, and they will have their effect.

Decide for yourself which text best suits your client or patient at any given time. You can also combine passages from different texts. It is not about using all ten hypnoses in sequence. It is a selection of possibilities.

I want to emphasize that books cannot replace therapy. Psychotherapy or other therapeutic treatments involve much more. A careful diagnosis is the necessary basis for deciding on the use of methods, including whether hypnosis or one of my texts should be used. Even in this case, preparatory discussions, follow-up discussions during the session, and of course, a therapeutic concept for the sequence of sessions and the content approaches are essential parts of therapy. This cannot and should not be achieved with a collection of texts.

In any case, I wish you much success in your work and I am pleased if my text templates can contribute in a small way.

Ingo Michael Simon

#1

Localized Chronic Pain

You want to reduce your pain, ideally even eliminate it completely ... ... Now is finally the time to let go of your pain ... ... You are mentally preparing yourself for this ... ... All your thoughts are focused on this goal because today you want to let go of your pain ... ... It's truly remarkable how quickly you can now bring this thought to the forefront ... ... You can do it ... ... You can do it today ... ... Your pain is becoming quieter ... ... your pain is becoming softer ... ... and a pleasant feeling is returning to your body ... ... If you now feel into your body, you will find many areas that feel good ... ... Focus on one such spot or area and feel how good it feels ... ... well done ... ... You are doing it exactly right ... ... You are entirely succeeding in now focusing only on the pleasant parts of your body ... ... You find a very pleasant spot in your body or a pleasant area ... ... Your whole body should feel like this ... ... Your entire body should feel this pleasant ... ... Today and every day ... ... Today and every day ... ... You decide to use the pleasant and light feeling of this area for your whole body ... ... To extend the relaxation and calmness of this area to your entire body ... ... You start this today and spread this feeling further in your body every day ... ... until your entire body feels this good ... ... You decide now to change your body ... ... to make it pain-free step by step ... ... Yes, you can do it, excellent ... ... You actually manage to make this decision with all your strength and to firmly establish that the pain-free zones of your body will fill your entire body with well-being ... ... well done ... ... very good, because that's how it actually works ... ... That's how it works ... ...

... ... You place a dial with ten levels where your body feels good ... ... a dial with ten levels ... ... As soon as you turn it, you can spread the pleasant feeling further ... ... with each level, with each number, the pleasant feeling spreads further in your body until your whole body feels like this spot that is so pleasant and above all completely pain-free ... ... Now place a dial at the good spot ... [It works better if you agree with the client on a specific spot that must be truly pain-free! Then directly address the spot ... Example: Now place a dial in your left leg ...] ...

Now focus on the dial ... ... and focus on exactly this point in your body ... ... When you start turning the dial, the well-being can spread step by step ... ... maybe with each number one or two centimeters ... ... that's enough ... ... and each time you turn it, you can gain two more centimeters of pain-free zone ... ... Now feel the pleasant sensation at the spot of the dial as intensely as possible ... ... The more you focus on this spot, the better it feels ... ... And now mentally prepare to turn the dial step by step, number by number ... ... I will help you with this ... ... So today you will already gain a few centimeters ... ... Take your time, because soon your whole body will be pain-free ... ... Maybe the painful area is far from the dial ... ... the better, because then the already pain-free part of your body can become even more relaxed and calm ... ... preparing even more to make your whole body pain-free ... ... With each number I mention, you turn the dial one step and spread the pleasant feeling of the healthy and pain-free relaxed spot in your body ... ... One ... ... Calmness and relaxation are spreading slowly ... ... [Wait for about ten seconds] ... ... Two ... ... you are actually succeeding ... ... At this very moment, you manage to extend the pleasant feeling from the good spot ... [Better directly address the agreed spot ... from your left leg ...] ... further ... ... Well done ... ... Three ... ... You extend the good feeling further ... ... [Wait for about ten seconds] ... ... Four ... ... The circle of pleasant feeling becomes another centimeter larger, maybe even two centimeters ... ... [Wait for about ten seconds] ... ... You are doing this excellently ... ... very, very well ... ... This is how your body will soon be pain-free ... ... Five ... ... It feels good ... ... really good ... ... [Wait for about ten seconds] ... ... Six ... ... The pleasant and above all completely pain-free feeling spreads ... ... Pain becomes smaller ... ... Pain fades step by step ... ... [Wait for about ten seconds] ... ... Seven ... ... You are doing very well ... ... You spread the well-being ... ... with each number a little further and soon over your entire body ... ... [Wait for about ten seconds] ... ... Eight ... ... Focus entirely on this pleasant area and feel how good this circle already feels ... ... [Wait for about ten seconds] ... ... Nine ... ... This is your pain-free circle that grows with each turn, with each number ... ... Today already a good piece, but soon all over your body, which will then finally feel completely good again ... ... completely good and pain-free ... ... pleasant and relaxed ...

… [Wait for about ten seconds] … … Ten … … Well done … … You already feel better … … When you imagine this circle around the good spot, around the dial, and look at it with your inner eye, the well-being at this spot, in this circle, becomes even more intense …

Your body imprints this very precisely. It knows that the pain-free circle, the circle of pleasant feeling, keeps expanding … … whenever you turn the dial … … So you can continue working on your liberation every day, you simply imagine turning the dial again, ten levels … … and with each level the pain-free circle expands further … … a few centimeters every day … … every day if you want … …

#2

Localized Chronic Pain

You want to reduce your pain, ideally even eliminate it completely ... ... Now is finally the time to let go of your pain ... ... You are mentally preparing yourself for this ... ... All your thoughts are focused on this goal because today you want to let go of your pain ... ... It's truly remarkable how quickly you can now bring this thought to the forefront ... ... You can do it ... ... You can do it today ... ... Your pain is becoming quieter ... ... your pain is becoming softer ... ... and a pleasant feeling is returning to your body ... ... If you now feel into your body, you will find many areas that feel good ... ... Focus on one such spot or area and feel how good it feels ... ... well done ... ... You are doing it exactly right ... ... You are entirely succeeding in now focusing only on the pleasant parts of your body ... ... You find a very pleasant spot in your body or a pleasant area ... ... Your whole body should feel like this ... ... Your entire body should feel this pleasant ... ... Today and every day ... ... Today and every day ... ... You decide to transform the pain in your body into exactly this pleasant feeling ... ... You start today and work every day to dissolve the pain ... ... until your whole body feels good again ... ... You decide now to change your body ... ... to make it pain-free step by step ... ... Yes, you can do it, excellent ... ... You actually manage to make this decision with all your strength and to firmly establish that the pain is now being reduced ... ... well done ... ... very good, because that's how it actually works ... ... That's how it works ... ...

... ... You place a dial with ten levels where your body has pain ... ... a dial with ten levels ... ... As soon as you turn it, you can reduce the pain ... ... with each level, with each number, you turn the pain down until your body is soon pleasantly and above all completely pain-free ... ... Now place a dial at the painful spot ... [Please directly address the painful spot or area ... Example: Now place a dial in your stomach ...] ... Now focus on the dial ... ... and focus on exactly this point in your body ... ... When you start turning the dial, you can actually reduce the pain ... ... with each number, you will feel it clearly ... ... Maybe you are already curious how clearly this will work ... ... and each time you turn it, you can reduce the pain further ... ... until they are completely gone ... ... The more you focus on this spot, the better it works ... ... And now mentally prepare to turn the dial step by step, number by number ... ... I will help you with this ... ... So today you will already reduce your pain ... ... Take your time because your pain will first become milder and then completely disappear ...

With each number I mention, you turn the dial one step and make the pain smaller ... ... One ... ... The pain is now becoming smaller, significantly smaller ... ... [Wait for about ten seconds] ... ... Yes ... ... maybe you already feel that the pain is decreasing or you will feel it in a few moments ... ... Two ... ... you are actually succeeding ... ... At this very moment, you manage to reduce the pain in ... [mention the painful spot/area] ... ... Well done ... ... Three ... ... You make it even smaller, turn it down ... ... [Wait for about ten seconds] ... ... Four ... ... The pain becomes smaller, you already feel better ... ... [Wait for about ten seconds] ... ... You are doing this excellently ... ... very, very well ... ... This is how your body will soon be pain-free ... ... Five ... ... It feels good ... ... really good ... ... [Wait for about ten seconds] ... ... Six ... ... Pain becomes smaller ... ... Pain fades step by step ... ... Your ... [mention the painful spot/area] ... already feels better, maybe a little better, maybe much better ... ... [Wait for about ten seconds] ... ... Seven ... ... You are doing very well ... ... You turn the pain down ... ... with each number a little further and soon they can disappear completely ... ... very soon ... ... [Wait for about ten seconds] ... ... Eight ... ... Focus entirely on this area of your body and feel how much better it already feels compared to before ... ... [Wait for about ten seconds] ... ... Nine ... ... Pain becomes quieter and quieter ... ... quieter and quieter ... ... You actually succeed ... ... Today already a good piece, but soon completely, so that your body will finally feel completely good again ... ... completely good and pain-free ... ... pleasant and relaxed ... ... [Wait for about ten seconds] ... ... Ten ... ... Well done ... ... You already feel better ... ... Enjoy today's success ... ... This is the beginning of freedom from pain ...

Your body imprints this very precisely. It knows that the dial in your imagination becomes the signal for reducing pain ... ... every time you turn the dial, your pain becomes smaller ... ... So you can continue working on your liberation from pain every day, you simply take some time and rest for yourself, lie down and imagine the dial ... ... Then you turn the dial again ... ... slowly ... ... step by step ... ... in ten levels ... ... and with each level, with each number, pain becomes quieter and quieter ... ... quieter and smaller every day ... ... every day if you want ... ... and I know you want it ... ... You want it more than anything else ... ...

#3

The following version of a hypnosis main part works with an anchor in the form of a "migraine magnet." This can be a flat, smooth stone, for example, a flat gemstone, or an animal shape cut out of foam rubber. I also like to use magnetic bracelets, which many people find pleasant. The effect of the migraine magnet has nothing to do with actual magnetism but with suggestively built associations. However, many clients subjectively believe in a more pronounced effect when actual magnetism is involved. And of course, it is also possible that the magnetic field provides support. I want to point out here that no magnet is needed for this hypnosis. An anchor is a trigger that is supposed to create a specific feeling or evoke a specific thought. We want to help the client use a "migraine magnet" to adjust faster to letting go of emerging migraine pain when they notice a migraine approaching in everyday life. Of course, it is actually about letting go or distancing the mental or psychological triggers of the migraine on an unconscious level. We discuss the procedure with our client before the session, who will then hold the migraine magnet to their head during the hypnosis. Please make sure to use this hypnosis only when the client does not have a headache. Once the client is accustomed to the procedure or the anchor is set up, they can use the procedure in everyday life for acute treatment.

You know the headaches you have had so often very well ... ... You know how they announce themselves and how they build up ... ... But now it's different ... ... Now, at this very moment, your head feels good ... ... A really nice feeling, so free and pleasant ... ... completely pain-free and calm ... ... It is often like this, but you want it to always be like this ... ... You want to prevent an oncoming migraine before it can even build up ... ... You want to avert an oncoming migraine before the pain can really take hold ... ... and if it does manage to break through, you want to pull the pain out of your head as quickly as possible ... ... You need a magnet to do that ... ... that simply pulls the pain out of your head ... ... and maybe you are surprised that this magnet actually exists ... ... You already have it in your hand ... ... You just need to activate it ... ... and that's exactly what you are doing here and today ... ... I will help you with that ... ... Now focus on the feeling of your head ... ... Right now, you have no pain ... ... no pain at all in your head ... ... But how does it feel? ... ... Feel your head now very consciously ... ... Feel how the cushion feels ... ... You feel the pillow under your head ... ... You can adjust the position of your head if you think it should be more comfortable ... ... if you think your head should lie softer or more stable or simply more comfortable ... ... Make yourself as comfortable as possible ... ... Then your head feels even better ... ... even much better ... ...

... ... Now imagine the word "pain" in your mind ... ... At the same time, you feel good because it's just a thought ... ... Imagine the word as if it is written in your head ... ... like letters that are in your head, forming the word "pain" ... ... well done ... ... that's very easy, comes very easily to you ... ... In your hand, you hold the migraine magnet ... ... This magnet is now learning how to relieve you of the pain ... ... It can be easier than you might have thought ... ... Guide your hand to your forehead and hold the migraine magnet against your forehead ... ... press it lightly with the palm of your hand against your forehead ... ... [Wait until the client holds the migraine magnet to their forehead. If they do not follow the prompt immediately, please prompt again more clearly! You can also help a little by guiding the client's hand a bit. Definitely announce this! ... I will help you and guide your hand a bit, well done, the rest you can do by yourself ...] ... well done ... ...

... ... Now imagine the letters of the word "pain" being drawn to the magnet ... ... First, the letter "P" is drawn ... ... It moves gently through your forehead and is absorbed and dissolved by the magnet ... ... Then the "a" follows ... ... The "a" of the word "pain" moves gently through the forehead and is absorbed and dissolved by the magnet ... ... Then follows the "i" ... ... The "i" of the word "pain" moves gently through the forehead and is absorbed and dissolved by the magnet ... ... Then follows the "n" ... ... The "n" of the word "pain" moves gently through the forehead and is absorbed and dissolved by the magnet ... ...

... ... Now feel once more the pleasant sensation in your head ... ... Your head feels pleasant and free ... ... no pain ... ... no pain ... ... Your head feels good ... ... Your magnet can do even more ... ... You can do even more ... ... Now imagine how it has often felt when the pain is coming on or even already there ... ... You can simply imagine it because you know how it can be ... ... Now you continue to feel good, but you imagine the pain in your head ... ... And then the magnet pulls the pain out of your head ... ... Step by step ... ... Piece by piece ... ... just like the letters of the word pain ... ... The word is an idea in your head, a thought ... ... maybe you know that the actual pain is also just an idea, a thought ... ... Your migraine magnet pulls the pain out of your head ... ... Imagine it, then your subconscious imprints it well ... ... well done, that's enough for now ... ... Everything is set up ...

Now you can help yourself every day in your everyday life ... ... whenever the pain starts to announce itself ... ... As soon as you notice the migraine approaching, take a few minutes of rest and press your migraine magnet against your forehead ... ... then imagine the word "pain" being drawn to your forehead letter by letter ... ... gently through the forehead and into the magnet that dissolves the letters ... ... and with each letter drawn out of your head, the oncoming migraine dissolves ... ... any pain that might be there is drawn out of your head letter by letter ... ... that's what your migraine magnet can do ... ... that's what you can do ... ... You succeed every day ... ... just as you succeeded today ... ...

#4

The following version of a hypnosis main part works with an anchor in the form of an "anti-pain cloth." This can be a simple silk cloth. An anchor is a trigger that is supposed to create a specific feeling or evoke a specific thought. We want to help the client use an "anti-pain cloth" to transfer a pain-free feeling from a healthy body part to a painful area. We discuss the procedure with our client before the session, and the "anti-pain cloth" is placed on a pain-free zone of their body that the client finds pleasant before the hypnosis begins. It should still be pleasant to the client if you, as the therapist, move the cloth during the trance and place it on the painful part of their body. If the painful area is in an intimate area or a place where the client does not want to be touched, you can agree with the client that they will place the cloth themselves and move it on your prompt during the trance. I generally prefer to let the client do as much as possible in such hypnosis sessions. Decide for yourself!

You want to soothe your pain, ideally eliminate it completely, so you can finally be pain-free again ... ... Now is finally the time to let go of your pain ... ... You are mentally preparing yourself for this ... ... All your thoughts are focused on this goal because you want to let go of your pain ... ... It is truly amazing how well you can now bring this thought so far forward that it can become reality ... ... You can do it ... ... You are doing it really well ... ... Your pain is becoming smaller ... ... your pain is becoming much smaller ... ... and a pleasant feeling is returning to your body ... ... If you now feel into your body, you will find many areas that feel good ... ... Especially the spot where the anti-pain cloth lies ... [Directly address the spot!] ... is completely pain-free ... ... Now focus on the spot where your anti-pain cloth lies and feel how good it feels there ... ... well done ... ... You are doing it exactly right ... ... You are entirely succeeding in now focusing only on this area of your body ... ... Your whole body should feel like this ... ... Your

entire body should feel this pleasant ... ... Today and every day ... ... Today and every day ... ... You decide to use the pleasant and light feeling of this body region for your whole body ... ... To transport the relaxation and calmness of this area to every part of your body ... ... This is actually possible ... ... You do it with the help of your anti-pain cloth ... ... You start today and transport as much of this good feeling as possible to the painful area of your body ... ... until it feels just as good ... ... You can do it ... ... You actually manage to make this decision with all your strength and to firmly establish that the feeling of being pain-free is transported with the help of the magic cloth ... ... You now focus on the position of the cloth ... ... The cloth is now connecting with your body ... ... The pleasant feeling of being pain-free ... ... of relaxation and calmness ... ... goes into this cloth as if it were your own skin ... ... The feeling that is under the cloth is now going into the cloth, which becomes a second skin ... ... The cloth on your body ... [Directly name the position ... The cloth on your leg ...] ... takes on the good feeling and stores it ... ... You are doing it right ... ... You have initiated this thought, and now it runs by itself ... ... Your anti-pain cloth becomes a feel-good cloth ... ... your wellness cloth ... ... a magic cloth that can transport this feeling to any part of your body ... ... The cloth on your body feels just as good as the spot where it lies ... ... and if you think your body should feel even better at this spot, then focus all your attention there ... ... Send all positive thoughts to where the magic cloth lies on your body ... ... well done, that is exactly right ... ... Now is the right time to transport this pleasant feeling, to simply bring it to the painful area because that will reduce the pain ... ... Maybe you wonder how quickly you will feel it when the cloth then lies like a new pain-free skin in the painful area of your body ... ... and maybe "painful area" will then no longer be the right term for it ...

[Now announce that you will pick up the cloth and place it in the painful area of the body. Of course, this text is formulated so that it is not tailored to a single pain variant. In practice, I always directly address the body part. Alternatively, instruct the client to move the cloth themselves. For this, they do not need to open their eyes; it works with closed eyes.]

Variant 1 (Therapist moves the cloth) ... ... I now pick up the magic feel-good cloth ... ... [Pick up the cloth] ... ... and place it in the painful area of your body ... ... [Place the cloth] ... ... like a second skin ... ... And now the pleasant feeling of the cloth flows right here into your body and soothes the pain ... ... The pain becomes smaller ... ... The cloth gives the well-being to your body ... ... Now this area can also feel better ... ... Pain becomes smaller ... ... Maybe you already feel it clearly ... ... maybe a bit later ...

Variant 2 (Client moves the cloth) ... ... Now pick up the magic feel-good cloth ... ... [Wait until the client picks up the cloth] ... ... and place it in the painful area of your body ... ... [Wait until the client places the cloth; if necessary, help!] ... ... It is like a second skin ... ... like a new skin ... ... And now the pleasant feeling of the cloth flows right here into your body and soothes the pain ... ... The pain becomes smaller ... ... The cloth gives the well-being to your body ... ... Now this area can also feel better ... ... Pain becomes smaller ... ... Maybe you already feel it clearly ... ... maybe a bit later ...

Let the pleasant feeling flow further into your body ... ... Enjoy the calmness and feel that it actually works ... ... maybe already very clearly ... ... maybe the cloth will also develop its full and strong effect a bit later ... ... Your body imprints this very precisely. It knows that the anti-pain cloth, your feel-good cloth, can transport the good feeling of freedom ... ... So you can continue working on your liberation from pain every day, you do it exactly as you did here and today ... ... You lie down and come to rest whenever you want, and place the magic cloth on a spot of your body that feels so good that you think your whole body should feel like this ... ... Then the feeling flows into the cloth, and you transport the cloth to the painful area ... ... Thus, you also transport the good feeling that can actually dissolve the pain ...

#5

You are here today to do something about your pain ... ... But often it is difficult to fight against something ... ... It is often much easier to fight for something ... ... So today you may end the fight against pain and begin your fight for freedom and relaxation ... ... for well-being ... ... Maybe you have noticed that there is no term for the opposite of pain ... ... Pain-free perhaps, but that is only a rejection of the term pain ... ... so let's say well-being and take this term as the state of being pain-free ... ... Far too often we cling to negative formulations, especially with pain so strongly that our language has not developed a real counterpart to it ... ... but today we call it well-being ... ... because well-being is completely incompatible with everything that pain entails ... ... So today is about your well-being ... ... If you could erase your pain, well-being would immediately set in ... ... and that is exactly possible ... ... You know that you can erase or at least numb pain with cooling ... ... If you then no longer feel it, you feel good again and can also free yourself internally from the pain ... ... because then you can think about something other than the pain ... ... Maybe you have burned yourself before and then cooled the painful spot with cold water and felt much better doing so ... ... But you do not need cold water ... ... all of that is also possible in your thoughts ... ... Thoughts and ideas work just as well, sometimes even faster than reality ... ... So now imagine some pictures that I offer you ... ... and each picture, each scene, you imagine as clearly and as intensely as possible ... ... At the same time, you adjust your body to develop the feeling of each picture and scene, to fully immerse yourself in it ...

... ... So let's go ... ... Imagine you are outside and it is raining ice-cold ... ... Ice-cold rain is pouring down from the sky like a downpour ... ... it is as if you were standing under an ice-cold shower ... ... The cold water flows over your skin, which becomes very cold and very numb ... ... The water is so cold that the sensation of your skin becomes almost numb ... ... ice-cold rain on your skin ... ... Imagine the rain ... ... Imagine standing naked in the rain and feeling the ice-cold water ... ... Your body absorbs this feeling ... ... Pain fades in the process ... ... Well-being can now spread ... ... a very pleasant well-being ... ... Then it is as if the water on your skin can wash away the pain, so it disappears forever ... ... It simply flows away with the cold water ... ... Then you see before your inner eye many penguins on an ice floe ... ... They huddle together on the cold floe ... ... around them is the ice-cold water of the polar sea ... ... and then they jump one after another into the icy water of the sea ... ... Hundreds of penguins jump into the cold water and feel perfectly at home in it ... ... Your body enters this feeling as if you were now jumping into the cold water and swimming after the penguins ... ... Your body absorbs this feeling ... ... Pain fades in the process ... ... Well-being can now spread ... ... a very pleasant well-being ... ... You already feel the cooling and soothing effect, and your body imprints this effect ... ... this connection of visual imagery and the actual feeling of relief ...

... ... Maybe you need more ... ... maybe you want to create another picture ... ... So imagine you are high in the mountains, and right in front of you is a mountain lake ... ... a small lake high in the mountains, with icy clear water ... ... You jump into the lake ... ... You imagine the icy water surrounding your whole body and cooling it ... ... It feels cool ... ... cold ... ... icy ... ... and indeed, with this imagination, you can feel it getting colder ... ... and that's good because it shows you that your body follows your ideas ... ... and cold water soothes pain ... ... This imagination also follows your body ... ... Maybe you have already noticed that your body has significantly less pain ... ... Your body cools and soothes the pain ... ... This works because you imagine being surrounded by cooling water ... ... It simply works ... ... You can even intensify the effect ... ... Just imagine it getting even colder because it starts to snow and because an icy winter wind blows over the mountains ... ... Then the water gets even colder ... ... maybe so cold that your body can hardly feel anything on the skin ... ... a feeling of numbness on the skin can arise ... ... and this feeling, which cannot allow any pain, then goes under the skin ... ... Pain fades ...

Your body imprints this ... ... Your whole organism imprints these images exactly ... ... cold rain ... ... penguins in the polar sea ... ... swimming in the mountain lake ... ... With all these images, you associate coldness that touches your skin and makes it numb ... ... Soothes pain because the sensation in the skin becomes duller ... ... You also associate that this feeling of numbness flows from the skin into the interior of your body and soothes pain there ... ... But you can do even more ... ... Every signal of relief is now also the signal for your organism to set in well-being ... ... to replace the pain with a pleasant feeling of relaxation ... ... You can use this every day for yourself

... ... You can recall these images with closed eyes and immediately relieve pain ... ... with the image of the ice-cold rain that immediately soothes pain ... ... with the image of the penguins in the polar sea that immediately soothes pain ... ... with the image of the mountain lake that immediately soothes pain ... ... Just imagine the images and then feel into your body and realize that pain actually fades ... ... just like now ... ...

#6

Pain is not just pain … … We can experience it very differently without physical change … … Sometimes the body hurts, and there is a clear reason for pain … … Sometimes physically perceived pain is hard to explain, or the intensity of the pain felt is higher than expected … … Just think back to your childhood … … Sometimes you fell or got hurt, and because you were playing, it only hurt a little … … maybe you didn't feel any pain at all while playing … … But later, when you calmed down, it did hurt … … Sometimes you were distracted or so full of excitement that you didn't notice the actual pain … … other times you focused so much on the pain or suffering that it hurt a lot … … You know this from adulthood too … … and also from emotions other than pain … … perhaps sadness or anger … … The more you thought about the reasons that made you sad or angry, the stronger the corresponding feeling was … … when you were distracted or focused on other things, different feelings were in the foreground … … and whenever you understood what made you sad or angry, when you worked through the underlying issues and resolved them, the feelings went away ... ... It's the same with pain ... ... if you understand or let go of what makes it so prominent and intense in your perception, the pain will also get smaller ... ... You can now start to let go of much of what makes you so attentive to the pain and thereby reduce the pain, maybe even soon dissolve or end it ... ... because your body will respond to the inner changes, to your letting go ...

... ... So now focus on your head and imagine that all the thoughts in your head are like small beads of different colors ... ... There are red beads for all the thoughts of fear ... ... You have often had fears and worries ... ... some fear has also influenced your pain ... ... sometimes even the thought of losing the pain can be frightening ... ... A part of the pain may have already become a routine that keeps you from changing and resolving other difficulties because the pain is so much in the foreground ... ... When you let go of fear, you can also let go of this part of fear ... ... You exhale the red beads with your next breaths ... ... They come out with your breath through your nose and fly through the room, expanding like soap bubbles ... ... and one by one they pop ... ... The fear goes away and is replaced by courage and strength … … Courage to look at and deal with everything in your life … … Courage to face all challenges … … Fear flies through the room like soap bubbles, and with each bubble that bursts, your fear dissolves … … whatever you are afraid of or could be afraid of, whether you know it or not … … You exhale your red fear thoughts … … You gather all the red thought beads in your head and exhale them as little red soap bubbles … … The red soap bubbles fly through the room and burst one by one, because you are letting go of the fear inside … … It has held you back, kept you from facing your conflicts and difficulties … … But now it is different … … Now you let go of fear, and with that, courage and strength grow in you … … Courage to look at and deal with everything in your life … … Courage to face all challenges … … The more red thoughts of fear and worry you exhale, the more courageous and stronger you become … … and the more you succeed in creating this image before your inner eye, seeing these red soap bubbles flying through the room, the more your body will also be able to let go of the pain … … make the pain smaller, because it is no longer so important … … So imagine the red thought beads in your head even more intensely and vividly … … Look at them before your inner eye and imagine how your breath carries them out of you ... ... well done ... ... You can do it ... ... You can imagine it ... ... You can build this picture ... ... You can actually see them ... ... and with that, you deeply understand that you can let go of fear because you decide to ... ... You can let go of the fear of confrontation and be brave ... ... You can let go of the fear of conflicts and be brave ... ... You can let go of the fear of losses and be brave ... ... You can let go of the fear of your own power and strength and be brave ... ... Watch the soap bubbles ... ... Observe how they fly through the room and especially how they burst ... ... one by one they burst ... ... Imagine standing beside yourself ... ... Stand beside the place where your body is lying/sitting and watch the red soap bubbles come out of your nose ... ... and burst one by one ... ... if you want, help them and make them burst with the tip of your index finger ... ... You can just pop them ... ... The fear goes away and is replaced by courage and strength ... ... Courage to look at and deal with everything in your life ... ... Courage to face all challenges ... ... and your pain suddenly becomes smaller and smaller ...

Your pain can indeed dissolve ... ... You can always make sure that what made your pain so prominent in your perception and interpretation dissolves like soap bubbles ... ... Just as you did today, you can imagine every day during a time of conscious breathing that the fear holding your pain comes out as soap bubbles from your nose and dissolves ... ... Fear bursts like soap bubbles ... ... Pain bursts like soap bubbles ... ... Pain bursts like soap bubbles ... ... Pain bursts like soap bubbles ...

#7

Ideomotorics refers to the phenomenon that our body follows our feelings and thoughts with movements. In everyday life, this following is shown as body posture, muscle tension, and movement patterns of a person, which naturally change with mood and thoughts. In trance, ideomotoric signals can be used to obtain information that the client cannot actively communicate. For example, the subconscious can answer questions with an agreed-upon finger signal. Of course, ideomotoric reactions can also be used suggestively, for example, with arm levitations and catalepsies. An approach like the one I use in the following text strengthens confidence in hypnosis and in one's own ability to change, thus promoting therapy.

For this, hold the client's arm at the wrist and pull it diagonally upwards without overstretching the arm. Test during the holding suggestion by giving slightly if the arm is already held cataleptically, and let go as soon as the catalepsy stands.

You want to let go of your pain and know that a large part of the pain arises in the thoughts ... ... in our dealing with the meaning of the pain ... ... in the thoughts about what limitations it means and how much it tortures and burdens us ... ... Then you also know that a constructive inner attitude helps to reduce the pain, even pain that has a physical cause ... ... You know this from the past ... ... If you cut your thumb, it hurts a lot when you are asked about it, when someone asks if it hurts ... ... But if you are distracted, you don't feel it at all ... ... It's similar with all pain, only it's not always so easy to distract yourself ... ... But if pain can be reduced by distraction, then it also works without distraction ... ... Your organism just has to apply the same principle, namely to direct your inner attention to other feelings ... ... Some changes are required for this, which are easier than you might think ... ... You want to reduce your pain ... ... or even switch it off ... ... Maybe you are wondering how it is possible to reduce pain so quickly ... ... You know it is possible, otherwise you wouldn't be here to get help with it ... ... I will show you how it works today ... ... You yourself can do it deep inside ... ... your inner self can do it ... ... and it can also show you as soon as it has done it ... ... For this, we will use your arm ... ... because your inner self ... ... your subconscious can show you with your arm that the pain is getting smaller, and you can then feel it immediately ... ...

[Now the client's arm is held by the therapist until the catalepsy stands. Discuss the procedure with the client before the session and always announce touches during the trance immediately. Always avoid any startle or defensive reactions!]

... ... I now take your wrist and hold your arm for you ... ... Just allow it ... ... Everything happens for your well-being ... ...

[Hold the client's arm at the wrist now and pull it diagonally upwards without overstretching the arm. Test during the subsequent holding suggestion by giving slightly if the arm is already held cataleptically and let go as soon as the catalepsy stands.]

... ... Now pay attention to your arm. It becomes firmer and firmer, as firm as an iron bar ... ... and feather-light ... ... it is very easy to hold the arm ... ... to hold it up as if it were held by an invisible balloon ... ... Your arm becomes firmer and firmer ... ... firmer and firmer, very firm and stable ... ... Your arm takes position and remains in exactly this position ... ... Your arm becomes stiff and firm and stays in exactly this position ... ... It is light and very firm ... ... Your arm is completely immobile and stiff ... ... completely immobile and stiff ... ... Your arm remains in exactly this position ... ... just like that ... ...

[Extend if necessary, if the arm is not held, which should happen quickly. For the client, the cataleptic state is not a subjective burden or strain. They feel as if the arm is holding itself.]

Your subconscious has already agreed to cooperate because it holds your arm for you ... ... because it is actually ready to significantly reduce your pain now ... ... Maybe you are already very curious about how much your subconscious can reduce the pain ... ... how clearly it can do it ... ... Now I give your subconscious the task of making your pain as small as possible and more is possible than you can imagine ... ... much more ... ... Pain becomes small and insignificant for you ... ... You will be surprised by the effect ... ... Your subconscious now adjusts to reduce the pain ... ... Your arm shows you how much your subconscious has already achieved ... ...

Your arm will now slowly become movable again and slowly sink to the surface ... ... This happens in exactly the same time your subconscious needs to significantly reduce your pain ... ... Your arm will only become movable and sink down when it is also possible to significantly reduce your pain at the same time ... ... only then will it be possible to make your arm movable and let it sink down ... ... and as soon as the arm reaches the surface, your pain is relieved as much as possible today ... ... As soon as your inner self is ready to reduce pain, your arm will become movable and sink to the surface ... ... as soon as your inner self is ready to let go of pain, your arm will become movable and sink to the surface ... ... It will happen ... ... It will happen today ... ...

[Wait until the arm sinks to the surface. This may take some time, but it can also go quickly. The speed does not matter for success. It reflects the determination of the will to change and any remaining doubts. Just let it run as it happens. If the arm does not move, help with the following or similar suggestions.]

Take your time ... ... Do it at your own speed ... ... at your own pace ... ...

As soon as the right moment is there, your arm will move ... ...

Surely today is the right day for it, then your arm will move right away ... ...

If today is not yet the right day, then your arm will not move today, but if today is the right day, it will move right away ... ...

... ... It works! ... ... Yes, that's good! ... ... Your body reduces the pain, and you can feel it ... ... You can feel it exactly ... ...

#8

The following hypnosis works with the connection between emotion and body. Since all feelings, just like thoughts, manifest in physical reactions—sometimes clearly, often subtly—focusing on body awareness and paying mindful attention to the body's signals can help solve problems. The client should be able to physically feel their deep-seated emotions and thus react more quickly to signs of emotional change. Suggestive techniques help to influence emotions by influencing body sensations because not only do feelings create body reactions, but targeted physical actions also affect sensations. For example, joy produces a smile, and conversely, a deliberate smile tends to brighten the inner mood. First, discuss with your client a spot on their body where you can press with a finger during hypnosis, and preferably also that you may lightly press into the center of the painful area with a finger of the other hand.

You have been in pain for a long time that you can no longer fully understand yourself ... ... They should actually have disappeared or be much less than you experience them ...... You have already thought a lot about why you feel this pain so strongly ...... You also know that our mental state can lead us to experience pain very differently ...... We could also say our psychological state or - and then it is even more precise - our emotionality ...... because it is very important how our emotional state is in a situation or over a longer period ...... Our emotions are our feelings ...... You might think that pain is also a feeling, but what is special is that many sensations we have are not really our inner feeling, but just mental interpretations ...... If our mind is convinced that a part of the body is injured or painful, it can actually feel that way ...... because we believe it ...... and because pain does not feel good at all, we believe even more and more strongly that it is actually there ...... We can hardly imagine that the pain is only in our thoughts then ...... and actually, it is not, because everything we physically feel is indeed in the body ...... It doesn't matter at all for our experience whether pain is measurable or detectable in the body ...... We feel it, and then it is there ...... Our body automatically and always reacts to our emotions, that is, our deep-seated feelings and to our thoughts ...... There is then an interesting connection ... ... On the one hand, our feelings and thoughts influence our body ... ... on the other hand, our body also influences our thoughts and feelings, can change them ... ... But not only thoughts and feelings can communicate with the body and influence it and vice versa, but different parts of the body can also connect with each other and influence each other ... ... change each other ... ... help each other ... ... A healthy part of the body can, for example, help an unhealthy part to get well again ... ... and a pain-free part can help a painful part to let go of the pain ... ... Maybe you knew that it's possible ... ... maybe you're wondering how quickly that can happen ... ... Maybe you're also wondering how quickly your body can manage to transfer the feeling from a pain-free part to a still painful part and thereby dissolve the pain ... ... That is indeed possible ... ... sometimes step by step ... ... but sometimes also with a big and clear step, so clearly that the pain simply stops ... ... All this is possible through body sensation and through thoughts ... ...

[Now place a finger on a pain-free spot or press lightly, then place a finger of the other hand in the center of the pain, if possible. Alternatively, the second finger can be placed at the edge of the pain zone. If neither is possible or suitable because the pain zone is in an intimate area or the client does not want to be touched, you can instruct the client to make the contact with their own hands. Simply discuss this before the session.]

... ... I now press with one finger on ... [Announce the agreed spot exactly before the session!] ... You now clearly feel my finger, and your body feels good here ... ... There is no pain here ... ... no pain at all ... ... Now consciously perceive the light pressure of my finger ... ... good ... ... Now I put another finger in your pain center ... ... I now press lightly on ... [Announce the agreed spot exactly before the session!] ... ... You now clearly feel my finger, and your body has (often) pain here ... ... There is (often) pain here ... ... Now consciously perceive the light pressure of my finger ... ... good ... ... and now I help your body to establish a connection from the pain-free to the painful spot ... ... This will lead to the information of the good feeling being transported to the pain center and reducing your pain there ... ... or ensuring that pain cannot come up so strongly anymore ... ... We transport the information of the good feeling to the pain center to reduce your pain now and for the future ... ...

... ... Focus on the finger that lies in the good zone ... [Apply noticeable pressure with the corresponding finger] ... ... And imagine a line leading to the pain zone ... ... [Apply noticeable pressure with the corresponding finger] ... ... Imagine a connection line between both points ... ... and imagine how information from the good zone repeatedly flows to the pain zone ... [Apply noticeable pressure with the corresponding finger] ... ... like a data transport from the pain-free spot [Apply noticeable pressure with the corresponding finger] ... to the pain center ... [Apply noticeable pressure with the corresponding finger] ... ...

... ... Imagine the connection line before your inner eye ... ... It works even better if you imagine an arrow connecting both points ... ... So, the information of the good feeling flows to the pain center, which feels better step by step ... ... Step by step, with each breath, the pain dissolves ... ... Maybe you can feel it already, or you will feel it in a few moments ... ... The clearer you can imagine the connection line or the connection arrow, the faster the good feeling is brought to the pain center ...

#9

Somatoform Pain

Today, you can take a special journey ... ... a journey that leads you deep into your own creativity and imagination ... ... The destination of this journey is yourself ... ... whatever you can experience and will experience always leads you back to yourself in the end ... ... Your body shows you the way there ... ... Simply follow the rhythm of your breathing and feel how it leaves your body with every breath ... ... Imagine that you could leave your body with the wind of your breath to embark on this journey ... ... This journey that takes you away from the limitations of space and time ... ... You leave your body now and go into the land of dreams ... ...

You find a wide path that leads across this land ... ... Full of trust, you wander along this path through the land of your dreams, and you discover a forest ... ... You follow the path further and simply walk into this forest ... ... You feel comfortable and go deeper and deeper into this forest ... ... You see old, mighty trees, and between the old trees, there are many smaller trees, even very small ones ... ... It is the forest of your thoughts, and all your thoughts are here. They are waiting for you here … … All the thoughts you have ever had are here … … and of course, all the thoughts you will have one day are here too … … And also, all the thoughts you could have at this very moment are here … … They are stored here for you … … Maybe you have a very clear and conscious thought at this moment … … perhaps a thought that expresses your will … … the will to let go of the pain … … and then you wonder how you can succeed in this … … what you can do to finally be free … … free from pain and finally have a good feeling again … … You have tried already … … You have also accepted that the pain comes from your thoughts, from mental entanglements, and not from your body … … You are looking for that one special thought that can help you the most today to end the pain … … You look deep into the forest and see large stones lying everywhere between the trees. They look like stone memorial plaques … … And that is exactly what they are … … Plaques that carry your thoughts … … On some, you find a word, like an engraving … … others may carry a short sentence or simply a symbol … … a special sign as a hint for you … … You might even discover a picture on some of them … … Then you just leave the wide path and walk right between the trees ... ... deeper and deeper into the forest, deeper and deeper into your own thoughts. And you keep seeing the memorial plaques of your own thoughts ... ... They are everywhere ... ... Some light up and show you a hint ... ... Others remain in the shadow, and you cannot read anything on them ... ... You go deeper and deeper into the forest because you are looking for that one thought ... ... for the decisive thought that can help you get out of the pain ... ... You can find that special thought today ... ... The thought that can help you the most today, that is the most important to end the pain right now and feel connected to yourself and others again ... ... You approach a very large memorial stone ... ... It is the largest and most beautiful far and wide ... ... On it, you find the thought of the moment ... ... the thought that can help you the most ... ... You get closer and closer ... ... Through the trees, a golden ray of light falls at this moment and bathes this stone in golden light ... ... It lights up, and you recognize the inscription ... ... You recognize the thought of the moment ... ... You can read it ... ... [wait for about half a minute, then continue reading] ... ... Maybe you expected this hint, or maybe it surprises you. But whatever it is - it is the most important thought ... ...

And if you cannot recognize it clearly, that is also perfectly fine because the thought is here ... ... Then you simply lay both hands on the stone and let the thought flow deep into your feeling and feel it ... ... You end the time of pain now, and step by step, it decreases ... ... The more you manage to listen to your own thoughts and moods, take them seriously, and become aware of them, the less pain you feel ... ... the faster it completely disappears ... ... You trust that this special thought will help you ... ... You know that the way to free yourself from your pain lies within yourself and that you can walk it again and again by becoming aware of your thoughts and feelings ... ... Then you walk back between the trees ... ... You carry the special thought within you ... ... You just let it be there, without having to understand it ... ... So, it does not matter at all whether you found a simple and clear thought or if it is a diffuse feeling that does not bring you an explanation ... ... It is not the explanation that helps you but the allowing ... ... The allowing of all thoughts ... ... and even more the allowing of all feelings ... ... You are already in the process of letting go of the pain ... ... You are already in the process ... ... And suddenly, you come to a new path ... ... It leads through the forest, but you had not seen it before ... ... This new path is your path ... ... This new path is your path ... ... You walk on this new path ... ... on the path of allowing your feelings ... ... on the path of accepting your feelings ... ... on the path that is your path ... ... the path of freeing yourself from pain ...

You come to the edge of the forest and walk out into the sun ... ... On a beautiful meadow, you find a comfortable place where you can rest ... ... You lie down and sink into your thoughts and dreams ... ... And you feel that the special thought you found spreads through you like a warm breeze ... ... Even if it might be an unpleasant thought, it will help you to continue letting go of your pain ... ... The thought and the feeling that belongs to it spread through you to inform every cell of your body about the thought ... ... about this inner truth that is so important and significant ... ... Then you think about how the land of dreams is deep inside you ... ... It has always been there ... ... I am only telling you about it ...

#10

Somatoform Pain

At night in our dreams, anything we can imagine is possible ... ... there are no limits, we don't need logic or reason ... ... Our feelings create the inner images and scenes that can help us learn more about ourselves ... ... understand more about ourselves ... ... be closer to ourselves ... ... But dreams do not belong only to the night and do not only show themselves in sleep ... ... Daydreams give us the same insight into our deepest inner self ... ... into the realm of the unconscious, which our reason cannot reach, but only our feeling can ... ... It is always our feelings that create our dreams ... ... You find every single dream in this special land within you ... ... in the land of dreams ... ... Your breath carries you there ... ... It blows your thoughts like a gentle wind into the land of dreams ... ... Now ... ...

You are standing on freshly plowed earth ... ... a field ready for sowing ... ... and in the middle of this freshly plowed earth lies a crystal ball ... ... in this sphere, which is so large that you can walk into it, you will find something you can understand in a single moment ... ... maybe this moment is very close today and you will experience it in the sphere ... ... or perhaps this one moment will come in one of the next few days, maybe it will come on any day in your life, and you will experience it again and again, recognizing and learning deeply within yourself ... ... Today, you want to understand how this happened ... ... how it could happen that such significant pain arose, even though your body is healthy ... ... So you walk up to this sphere and look inside ... ... Inside, there is a couch like at a doctor's or in a hospital ... ... With a large step, you enter the sphere ... ... You lie down on the couch and look at the wall of the sphere that arches over you ... ... and slowly, gradually, images appear on the wall of the sphere ... ... images showing you scenes and impressions from a time long before your pain ... ... You focus on the spot or area of your body that has been affected by the pain for so long, and you consider what feeling might be stored in that exact spot of your body ... ... You continue to focus and look up, seeing images from the time when the feeling in this part of your body originated ... ... Perhaps images from the recent past ... ... a few years ago ... ... or from a very long time ago, who knows ... ... Just let the images be there, whatever they show you ... ... maybe you see events, maybe also people ... ... They do not show you who caused the pain or how exactly it came about ... ... but they take you to the time when it arose and grew ... ... You immerse yourself in the images ... ... Maybe there are many images ... ... maybe just a few ... ... possibly only a single, very special image or a scene from your memory ... ... a situation or a person ... ... Just allow whatever you see ... ... even if a memory comes to mind that took place at a time when the pain was already there ... ... and even if you cannot recognize anything or no thought comes to mind, the images are already here in the sphere ... ... Then simply feel into the part of your body that is affected by the pain ... ... and feel what your body feels there now, in this exact moment ... ... You don't have to give this feeling a name ... ... You don't have to describe it or label it ... ... don't even have to find a designation for it, because that would already be an interpretation and thus a judgment ... ... But for your feelings, there are neither judgments nor interpretations ... ... Feelings can neither be wrong nor bad ... ... They are just as they are ... ...

There is a sensation in your body that you can perceive, that is enough ... ... Perceive this sensation now ... ... At that time, the circumstances weakened you and drained your strength, at that time it couldn't happen in any other way than to react with pain ... ... physical pain expressing your emotional pain ... ... because you couldn't perceive your own feelings unfiltered ... ... You had believed that you had to hide them ... ... perhaps paid more attention to what feelings were expected of you ... ... or what you allowed yourself to feel ... ... and these have a lot to do with what feelings were imposed on you as the desired ones ... ... Today, you might be able to feel your feelings from back then better, but maybe you are not sure what your current sensations are ... ... Don't worry, everything is alright ... ... It's not about understanding or recognizing anything with your mind, that would be the wrong path or at least a very uncertain one ... ... The necessary thing happens deep in the world of your feelings at this very moment ... ... simply by being here and allowing the images and memories ... ... and accepting every feeling that may arise in you ... ... without judgment ... ... without guilt ... ... completely relaxed in your imagination ... ... Once you learned to react with pain ... ... Your body had decided it that way to send you a signal ... ... a signal showing you that you had suffered deeply inside ... ... perhaps still suffer ... ... But now you can take care of it ... ... Your body can now stop sending you this signal ... ... You don't need this message anymore ... ...

Now you can let go ... ... you can let go of your physical pain because you no longer need it ... ... You know that it is inner pain ... ... your body only signaled to you that it exists ... ... But much more has happened ... ... While you were in your thoughts and images, your deep inner self, your subconscious, has already learned to now tackle the inner problems ... ... Thus, the physical pain becomes unnecessary ... ... Then you think about how the land of dreams is deep within you ... ... It has always been there ... ... I am just telling you about it ...

Distribution, publication, and copying in any form are prohibited and subject to damages.

Overview of All Titles in the Series "Ten Hypnoses"

Volume 1: Smoking Cessation
Volume 2: Anxiety and Restlessness
Volume 3: Burnout
Volume 4: Reducing Overweight
Volume 5: Coping with the Past
Volume 6: Suicidal Thoughts and Attempts
Volume 7: Psycho-Oncology
Volume 8: Obsessions and Tics
Volume 9: Self-Confidence and Decision-Making
Volume 10: Grief Work
Volume 11: Psychosomatics
Volume 12: Chronic Pain
Volume 13: Depressive Thoughts
Volume 14: Panic Attacks
Volume 15: Domestic Violence, Victim Support
Volume 16: Post-Traumatic Stress
Volume 17: Exam Anxiety and Stage Fright
Volume 18: Anti-Violence Training, Offender Support
Volume 19: Addiction Tendencies
Volume 20: Social Phobia and Fear of Contact
Volume 21: Nail Biting
Volume 22: Self-Awareness and Self-Love
Volume 23: Teeth Grinding and Night Clenching
Volume 24: Feelings of Guilt
Volume 25: Fear in Crowds
Volume 26: Fear of Flying, Aviophobia
Volume 27: Fear in Enclosed Spaces, Claustrophobia
Volume 28: Tinnitus, Ear Noises
Volume 29: Fear of Heights
Volume 30: Neurodermatitis

Copying, publishing, and sharing with third parties are only permitted with the written consent of the author. Please observe the notes on copyright and usage.

Volume 31: Finding Inner Balance
Volume 32: Overcoming Loneliness
Volume 33: Fear of Illness, Hypochondria
Volume 34: Anticipatory Anxiety, Fear of Fear
Volume 35: Jealousy in Relationships
Volume 36: Driving Anxiety
Volume 37: New Start after Separation
Volume 38: Fear of Injections
Volume 39: Heart Anxiety Neurosis
Volume 40: Overcoming Resentment and Anger
Volume 41: Resolving Blockages and Positive Thinking
Volume 42: Stress Reduction, Stress Management
Volume 43: Body Relaxation
Volume 44: Deep Relaxation
Volume 45: Fear of the Dark
Volume 46: Falling Asleep and Staying Asleep
Volume 47: Compulsive Buying
Volume 48: Restless Legs Syndrome
Volume 49: Bulimia
Volume 50: Anorexia
Volume 51: Overcoming Nightmares
Volume 52: Imagined Deformity
Volume 53: Overcoming Distrust, Finding Trust
Volume 54: Processing Failures
Volume 55: Humiliation, Emotional Hurt
Volume 56: Distressing Compassion, Vicarious Suffering
Volume 57: Self-Forgiveness
Volume 58: Self-Awareness, Self-Confidence
Volume 59: Saying No
Volume 60: Assertiveness
Volume 61: Setting Boundaries and Self-Assertion
Volume 62: Decision-Making Ability

Volume 63: Success Orientation
Volume 64: Ruminating, Circular Thinking
Volume 65: Accepting Pregnancy
Volume 66: Birth Preparation
Volume 67: Spiritual Opening
Volume 68: Joy of Life and Inner Lightness
Volume 69: Patience and Inner Peace
Volume 70: Fibromyalgia and Rheumatism
Volume 71: Irritable Bowel Syndrome, Crohn's Disease
Volume 72: Fear of Nausea, Emetophobia
Volume 73: Stuttering and Cluttering, Speech Flow Disorders
Volume 74: Concentration and Knowledge Anchoring
Volume 75: Vitality and Spontaneity
Volume 76: Searching for Meaning and Finding Goals
Volume 77: Life Crises, Life Events
Volume 78: Workaholism, Goal Obsession
Volume 79: Helper Syndrome, Helpless Helpers
Volume 80: Medication Abuse
Volume 81: Gambling Addiction
Volume 82: Internet Addiction, Smartphone Addiction
Volume 83: Hoarding Disorder, Compulsive Collecting
Volume 84: Conspiracy Thoughts, Overvalued Ideas
Volume 85: Fear of Operations and Treatments
Volume 86: Fear of Aging
Volume 87: Travel Anxiety
Volume 88: Anxiety When Urinating, Paruresis
Volume 89: Fear of Intimacy and Togetherness
Volume 90: Fear of Blushing
Volume 91: Coming Out in Homosexuality
Volume 92: Charisma Training
Volume 93: Migraines and Chronic Headaches
Volume 94: Overcoming Allergies, Bronchial Asthma

Volume 95: Normalizing Blood Pressure
Volume 96: Compulsive Perfectionism
Volume 97: Sports Hypnosis, Motivation
Volume 98: Sports Hypnosis, Performance Enhancement
Volume 99: Determination and Focus
Volume 100: Encountering the Inner Child
Volume 101: Cravings, Binge Eating
Volume 102: Stimulating Metabolism
Volume 103: Bipolar Mood Swings
Volume 104: Borderline, Identity Crises
Volume 105: Hypomania, Euphoria, Mania
Volume 106: Restlessness, Agitation
Volume 107: Nervous Breakdown
Volume 108: Adjustment Disorders
Volume 109: Self-Alienation, Depersonalization
Volume 110: Ending Self-Pity
Volume 111: Primary Gain of Illness
Volume 112: Secondary Gain of Illness
Volume 113: Bullying, Victim Support
Volume 114: Letting Go of Envy and Jealousy
Volume 115: Fear of Spiders, Arachnophobia
Volume 116: Fear of Dogs or Cats
Volume 117: Fear of Strangers, Xenophobia
Volume 118: Excessive Worries, Generalized Anxiety
Volume 119: Strengthening Sense of Responsibility
Volume 120: Unrequited Love, Heartache
Volume 121: Work-Life Balance
Volume 122: Letting Go of Unattainable Goals
Volume 123: Allowing and Accepting Help
Volume 124: Letting Go of Adult Children
Volume 125: Tourette Syndrome
Volume 126: Life Changes and New Starts

Volume 127: Accepting Life in a Wheelchair
Volume 128: Understanding and Overcoming Homesickness
Volume 129: Understanding and Overcoming Wanderlust
Volume 130: Dizziness, Meniere's Disease
Volume 131: Overcoming Aggression
Volume 132: Cutting and Self-Harm
Volume 133: Hair Pulling, Trichotillomania
Volume 134: Postpartum Depression
Volume 135: For Relatives of Dementia Patients
Volume 136: Self-Harm, Artificial Disorders
Volume 137: Activating Self-Healing Powers
Volume 138: Preventing Depression Relapse
Volume 139: Reactive Psychoses, Follow-Up
Volume 140: Obsessive Thoughts and Impulses
Volume 141: Compulsive Checking
Volume 142: Compulsive Counting, Symmetry Obsession
Volume 143: Compulsive Washing, Cleanliness Obsession
Volume 144: Compulsive Questioning
Volume 145: Dissociative Paralysis
Volume 146: Phantom Pain
Volume 147: Overcoming Complaining
Volume 148: Hay Fever, Pollen Allergy
Volume 149: Sexual Abuse, Victim Support
Volume 150: Standing Strong Against Sexism, #metoo
Volume 151: Binge Eating
Volume 152: Overcoming Thoughts of Revenge
Volume 153: Detachment from the Aggressor, Stockholm Syndrome
Volume 154: Courage to Separate
Volume 155: Chronic Fatigue, Exhaustion
Volume 156: Fear of the Future, Existential Anxiety
Volume 157: Excessive Worry About Children
Volume 158: Fear of Failure

Volume 159: Ending Distrust and Control
Volume 160: Dejection, Dysphoria
Volume 161: Boreout, Chronic Boredom
Volume 162: Bipolar Disorders, Relapse Prevention
Volume 163: Mania, Relapse Prevention
Volume 164: Nihilism, Feelings of Worthlessness
Volume 165: Thumb Sucking
Volume 166: Being Brave
Volume 167: Being Proud
Volume 168: Overcoming Shyness
Volume 169: Being Able to Delegate Responsibility
Volume 170: Being Able to Show Emotions
Volume 171: Letting Go of Guilt, Victim Support
Volume 172: Processing Guilt, Offender Support
Volume 173: Mood Swings, Cyclothymia
Volume 174: Lack of Drive, Vital Sadness
Volume 175: Hearing Voices with Reality Reference
Volume 176: Confident Communication
Volume 177: Standing Up for Oneself
Volume 178: Taking New Paths
Volume 179: Confident Job Application
Volume 180: No Longer Being Taken Advantage Of
Volume 181: End of Submissiveness
Volume 182: Depressive Numbness
Volume 183: Mood Drops, Affective Incontinence
Volume 184: Mood Instability
Volume 185: Somatoform Disorders
Volume 186: Stomach Ulcer, Psychosomatic
Volume 187: Accepting Amputation
Volume 188: Overcoming and Letting Go of Hatred
Volume 189: Ending Accusations
Volume 190: Allowing Tears, Being Able to Cry

Volume 191: Finding and Sorting Repressed Feelings
Volume 192: Somatoform Pain
Volume 193: Living Autonomously
Volume 194: Anhedonia, Joylessness
Volume 195: Persistent Sadness
Volume 196: Obesity, Food Addiction
Volume 197: Parents of Abused Children
Volume 198: Letting Go and Letting Be
Volume 199: Childhood Sexual Abuse
Volume 200: Fear of Loss

www.ingramcontent.com/pod-product-compliance
Lightning Source LLC
Chambersburg PA
CBHW030459220526
45464CB00006B/2575